60+ AND GOING STRONG:
Walking to a Healthier You...

Janice M. Lauderdale

Published:

Los Angeles, CA

Copyright April 2015

60+ and Going Strong: Walking to a Healthier You...
by Janice M. Lauderdale
janmarielauderdale@gmail.com
http://lauderdaleliteraryworks.com/65soaringprofits
http://indiebestwriters.com

Janice M. Lauderdale
Published in USA

Table of Contents

If You Are Alive; You're Getting Older
A Hearty Endorsement... 4

Introduction 5

Step 1: Facing the Facts.. 6

Step 2: Taking Control 13

Step 3: If a Little Bit is Good – More is Better! 17

Step 4: Revolutionize Your Life by Walking 21

Step 5: Good Walking Techniques are Key....................................27

Step 6: Defying the Odds 30

Step 7: One Courageous Moment 32

BIOGRAPHY Janice M. Lauderdale.. 34

If You Are Alive; You're Getting Older
A Hearty Endorsement

We are all getting older and if quality of life is severely compromised it poses a problem. Training and assisting the elderly require a special skill set to do. When one is forced into caring for an elderly loved one that he or she isn't prepared for, that becomes the problem.

This book picks up where laymen's knowledge of the elderly falls off. It is loaded with insightful tips, and is a highly recommended read for every baby boomer, senior, and those who care for and about them. Janice does a great job of exposing fallacies about the elderly lifestyle that could help millions of seniors, baby boomers, and their loved ones.

Ryan Lauderdale

Owner of Rypen Fitness Solutions

Nike Master Trainer

Rypenfitness.com

Introduction

An introduction is appropriate here, please allow me!

My name is Janice Lauderdale; I've been married to my husband Dennis for 40 years. You might be saying, okay, we got your name and what's the point? Well, my name is far less important than my journey from sickness, debilitation, two bad knees, 50 pounds overweight, and tiredness all the time. I want to share with you how you can overcome all that I overcame. We have two adult children and live good retirement years in Los Angeles.

Well, that was so until one morning when I woke up with two sharp pains running through my legs. I almost buckled to the floor. I was devastated, but I overcame it.

I promise you that if you follow the 7 Steps outlined in my book, I know that you will walk again, pain free, just as I am walking. No great walking guru can promise what they have not lived. My journey is real, and I ask you to come along with me, do what I did, and see your life change, as mine changed.

Step 1:
Facing the Facts

I had a serious problem and was determined to do something about it. As a consequence of the devastation I went through a few years earlier, it seemed that my body and heart were forever changed. I was 50 pounds overweight and climbing. No, let's be real. I had blown up as big as a house. I was now taking blood pressure medication daily and my entire appearance looked like one big blimp. I was almost unrecognizable, even to myself!

The pain I went through settled deep inside me. As a matter of fact, I didn't think that anything I had faced in life could rival the agony I was now facing— filing taxes, keeping up with family business concerns, banking and taking care of our household. I just wanted to go and hide from tiredness and stress. I almost resigned myself to accepting this state as my new normal. Every day felt more difficult, more challenging, and absolutely depleting. My situation was a deep dark hole that only got deeper and darker with each passing day.

I had hoped the conclusion of the court hearing with my brother concerning his abuse of and theft from my elderly aunt would ease my pain. Let me tell you about that—my aunt, 87 years old, ended up with my brother who stripped her of her life's savings and tried to take her fully-paid-for house by bogus trust.

I attempted to move forward, but it seemed that for every step I took forward, I took two backwards, gaining no ground. I mostly felt as if I were on the losing end. My entire life began to unravel because I couldn't seem to pry my emotions from past betrayal and pain. I simply could not wrap my brain around the fact that my brother betrayed my aunt. The thought of it always brought tears. Waking up each morning was one continuous day of devastation.

I cried way too much, but the tears were cleansing and that was exactly what I needed. I wanted and deserved all of that betrayal to be washed from my mind. Yet, my raw emotions had to be revealed regardless of the scorn directed at me by gallery bystanders. Mine was a life that had to be put back together. With the sadness in my heart as well as excruciating pain in my knees, I was determined to move to a new place in life.

Healing and wholeness are two of the most powerful entities in life. I wondered how I could get better, and an opportunity presented itself that very day. It allowed me to get rid of that toxic stuff that was eating me alive. So, I wrote a book about the betrayal of my brother with my aunt. I became a published author—*"Wealth of the Wicked: an American Tragedy of Elderly Abuse."*

Writing my book became one of the best forms of therapy for me. It was so cathartic. I shared my story with the world, and found so many matching stories involving elderly abuse. Still I wasn't healed. I took pain pills that had more side effects than cures. I would always ask the doctor, "What are the side effects?"

The side effects seemed more harmful than the sickness. I sighed. I didn't like it at all.

After writing my book, I began to see life through my same old frames but with new lenses. I was making a comeback. I hadn't smiled for a long time, but now, I began to see the humor in life again. And it all felt good!

I was seriously moving to a new plateau and enjoying what I saw and felt. I seriously took on a walking exercise routine, which led to 20 miles a week. I was sore but began to feel revived. In case you're wondering whether I started out at 20 miles a week; no, I did not. I started at a one mile hike for a year. Then I moved up to two, then three, then a four mile walk. Looking back and wondering how that happened, I would say the biggest contributor was consistency. There were days when I didn't want to go. I had enough excuses to share with anyone who passed by. I had heart-to-heart conversations on the long-range benefits awaiting me, but the voice of reason always prevailed. I was deeply invested in my four-mile a day walk. I felt so invigorated, so alive, and so determined. There was nothing and nobody that could stop me.

Nineteen ninety-nine was a year that is etched in my memory and not for all good reasons. I felt great, and I might add that I didn't look so bad either. So, on one sunny morning with a world of hope in my heart, I set out on my 4-mile walk. I had only walked about 500 feet and something dreadful happened that would chart the course of my life for many years to come. An excruciating, sharp pain, ripped through both my knees with reckless abandon, unrelenting. Vicious. I couldn't figure it out. But, one thing was sure: I couldn't walk. I turned around and managed to hobble and drag my way back home.

After seeing my doctor and being diagnosed with bilateral knee degenerative arthritis, I knew my life would take a different form, not one I was proud to claim. For many years I was in and out of the doctor's office desperately seeking a solution for the new calamity that had just put my life in a tailspin. I participated in clinical trials which included the testing of new medications, all to no avail. I was desperate for relief, and my doctor did what doctors do: gave me more pain pills. After three months, they sent me to physical therapy with marginal benefits.

After one of my doctor's appointments, along with my medical prescription, I was handed a companion that would too soon become a good friend– a non-descript black single-point cane. And, I said to myself, "what am I supposed to do with this little stick"

Well, that cane became a real buddy, going with me everywhere. I imagined American Express' signature warning, "Don't leave home without it." Well, that's exactly how I felt about my new best-bud, my cane. It went with me everywhere.

I tried to settle into my new routine, but with the onset of ever increasing pain, it became more difficult to walk across the room. And, oh did I forget to mention that my condition was made worse because I also had the sudden onset of sciatica. If you've never experienced this malady, it might be a little difficult for you to relate. But, if you have, then you know exactly what I mean when I say it was some of the worse pain I ever had, right up there with childbirth. It was horrible. Standing, walking, sitting were all too difficult for me. I was a mess! I felt hopeless and helpless, until…

My son, Ryan who is a strength and conditioning coach, and might I add a very good one, looked at me one day while I sat at the kitchen table, as if he were studying me. The look wasn't good. He knew me as a person who was a fighter and not one to succumb to life's pitfalls.

"Mom, you need to exercise that away," he said.

I agreed with him and he started me on a training program. It was not a walk in the park, but absolutely intense. He'd have me to lie on the floor and one of the exercises involved twisting my reluctant body like a pretzel. I screamed because the pain felt like I would die. And, you know what? He was unimpressed and unmoved. He had heard those piercing sounds so many times before with his clients.

"But, I'm your mother!"

"Mom, you're only making it harder on yourself."

"That's easy for you to say."

"You'll be all right."

Under Ryan's tutelage, here's what my daily routine turned out to be:

- I joined a water aerobics class at my local park 3 times a week. For those who have a fear of water, remember, water aerobics does not involve any submerging of your head in the water. The benefits are immeasurable.
- I followed the exercise plan Ryan laid out.
- I rode my recumbent bike. A recumbent bike takes pressure off my knees, which is what I needed.
- I gave serious consideration to losing weight.
- I tried to maintain a good mental attitude, the key to my success.

I knew I should have had a more proactive attitude toward my health for a long time. Instead, I lived with agonizing pain in my knees and my back while I wondered if it was possible to ever be free of pain. I was so invested in providing caregiving for my elderly aunt that I couldn't entertain the thought of knee surgery. That kind of action would require a serious commitment to my post-surgery.

After many years of devotion to my aunt, she passed away in 2005. After a period of mourning, I decided to make an investment in my health that had been tabled for many years. Soon I discovered that the right time had not yet come. I was called into the new duty of caregiving for my own aging mother.

With excruciating pain in my cartilage-less knees, I was there for mom. Isn't that what good children do? I believe one of the worse situations in a person's life is looking backwards, wondering what if. Thankfully, I wasn't tormented by the time I spent helping my aunt, or caring for my mom.

In life, it's not always clear why we go through such trauma, but I have no doubt that I have endured much to provide some semblance of hope for those who find themselves in need of my assistance. Since becoming my aunt and mother's aide, I learned much and have become a passionate advocate on behalf of those 60+.

I studied what would make me live my boomer years with organic health. Walking daily is a key to organic wellness. You don't need a buddy. There are no side effects, no medications.

Sometimes we are astonished by what we see in ourselves. Perhaps, when you see someone going through a hard situation, you say to yourself, "I'd never be able to handle that."

Unfortunately you won't know until you're confronted with something similar or worse. But the greater you will appear when you come face to face with life and death. You will find yourself gearing up to be the conqueror that you really are. We are privileged to go into battle on someone else's behalf, or you fight through your own battle. The best in us shines like the breaking of a new dawn. It's the best feeling ever!

My physical condition began to deteriorate rapidly and I was no longer able to do anything for my mother whose health also took a serious decline. My sister took leave from her job in Atlanta and came home to care for her. What a relief! I had someone to trade off days in caring for mom. What we didn't know was that those were her last days. I was a mixed bag of emotions, thankful and sad at the same time. I was going to have my surgery but thoughts of my mother's health decline always stopped me from taking action. Now I was going to do it.

Finally on September 12, 2012, with bags packed, my husband Dennis and I headed to Kaiser Hospital in Harbor City for my double knee replacements. I had decided I would have both surgeries at the same time; even though I had been advised against it. My doctor prepared me for what to expect.

He told me how difficult it would be to have one knee replaced but two at one time would be rare. He even told me how concerned he was about my post-surgical course. I didn't back down because I knew I would do everything possible to get my life back. Now I am going to show how you too can get organic health without damaging your body with the side effects of taking pill after pill.

Step 2:
Taking Control

After a successful surgery, I was warned about being diligent in following therapy. "Don't do it, or half do it, and you'll be a cripple for the rest of your life," the doctor warned.

I was sent to rehab for a week and released early because of my set determination that produced tremendous progress. I remember walking down a very long hallway with the physical therapist in tow, and when I looked around I had left him in the dust. I was making a miraculous recovery.

In one week, I was released home. It was there that the very hard work began. But, I was determined to get my health back and to feeling well without pills, without the awful side effects the pain medication could have on my body. I was ready for the hard work. Most of the hospital equipment I was sent home with is still in the box.

I was ecstatic about my progress. When I had my first post-surgical appointment with my doctor, I asked, "Are you still worried about me?"

"No, not at all. You're doing miraculously well."

One week after my release from rehab I went to see my mother with my lifetime bow legs straightened. She was so happy for me. Just above a whisper, smiling from ear to ear, she said, "Come around here and let me see those straight legs."

What a precious moment, even though her physical condition had deteriorated more than she or the family knew. On September 30, 2012, one week after my return home, she passed into heaven. My knees were still hurting, but the pain in my heart from losing my mother took its place. She was not only my mother but my dearest friend!

Only a week after her memorial service and burial, I tackled my post-surgical program again. I was relentless with my exercises. If the therapist advised that I do three repetitions, I did six. I needed to be focused, and I was. After only one month, I was told that the range of motion in my knees was normal. I had heard far too many tragic stories of people who had joint replacement surgery and were crippled for life. I felt totally strong and elated.

My mom was one of my biggest cheerleaders. Pleasant thoughts of her overflowed my heart as I mounted those steps without the assistance of my cane, to speak a word in her memory. She would have been so proud. That's who she was.

I wondered if those people in the stats were as invested in doing those exercises as I was. How serious were they about WALKING? That's the key. Was it painful? Yes. But I knew I had to push past the excruciating pain, and I did. Each day that I performed those exercises, I noticed less and less pain. It even became tolerable.

I took the pain medication prescribed but for no longer than necessary. I wanted to make sure I was getting better because of my efforts and not because I was covering the agony by popping pills every day. I can truthfully say I did some things very well, and now I can see the results of my labor.

My post-operative exercise routine consisted of the following:

1. **Quadriceps Sets**
   - Tighten your thigh muscle. Try to straighten your knee. Hold for 5 to 10 seconds.

- Repeat this exercise approximately 10 times during a two minute period, rest one minute and repeat. Continue until your thigh feels fatigued.

2. **Straight Leg Raises**

   - Tighten the thigh muscle with your knee fully straightened on the bed, as with the Quad set. Lift your leg several inches. Hold for five to 10 seconds. Slowly lower.

   - Repeat until your thigh feels fatigued.

   - You can also do the leg raises while sitting. Fully tighten your thigh muscle and hold your knee fully straightened with your leg unsupported. Repeat as above. Continue these exercises periodically until full straightening returns to your thigh.

3. **Ankle Pumps**

   - Move your foot up and down rhythmically by contracting the calf and shin muscles. Perform the exercise periodically for two to three minutes, two or three times an hour.

4. **Knee Straightening Exercises**

   - Place a small rolled towel just above your heel so that it is not touching the bed. Tighten your thigh. Try to fully straighten your knee and to touch the back of your knee to the bed. Hold fully straightened for 5 to 10 seconds.

   - Repeat until your thigh feels fatigued.

5. **Bed-Supported Knee Bends**

   - Bend your knee as much as possible while sliding your foot on the bed. Hold your knee in a maximally bent position for 5 to 10 seconds and then straighten.

- Repeat several times until your leg feels fatigued or until you can completely bend your knee.

6. **Sitting Supported Knee Bends**

- While sitting at bedside or in a chair with your thigh supported, place your foot behind the heel of your operated knee for support. Slowly bend your knee as far as you can. Hold your knee in this position for 5 to 10 seconds.

- Repeat several times until your leg feels fatigued or until you can completely bend your knee.

www.orthoinfo.aaos.org

In April of 2013, I felt the overwhelming urge to go for a walk. I was ready and willing to give it a try. I started out walking in my neighborhood for approximately 20 minutes and in the next 3 weeks I was walking a mile. Yay! I felt an energy I hadn't felt in years. I kept extending my milestones a mile, then another mile. I extended my walk time to 40 minutes or about 2.5 miles. I was on a roll – unstoppable. I was feeling real well.

Step 3:
If a Little Bit is Good –
More is Better!

By June of 2013, I felt like superwoman ready to conquer the world. I extended my walk time to 1 hour and 10 minutes, which translated into about 3.4 miles.

Once again, I challenged myself to kick into another gear. On November 8, 2013, I convinced myself that I was ready for the next step, and walked for 4 miles. I walked 4 miles a day for no less than 5 days a week and sometimes 6 until November 2014 when the challenge was on again. I said to myself, self you can do a little more. And I was right.

November 2014, I took the challenge to another level and increased my walking time to 5 miles a day; that's right, 5 miles a day for at least 5 days and often 6 days a week. Not bad for a 67 year-old with simultaneous double knee surgeries! I see a pattern of behavior taking place in me. The more I challenge myself, the more I am challenged.

A high point of my progress with my health began in February 2014 when I participated in the Redondo Beach Super Bowl 5k Run/Walk. I had prepared myself and felt good about competing in the race. I finished. What an accomplishment. Super Woman, indeed!

Two thousand fifteen has been another milestone in my life. In January, I answered the challenge again. I am now walking 6 miles 5 days a week and sometimes 6 days. The benefits from walking have been tremendous. I've lost a significant amount of weight and feel great. Additionally, it takes me approximately 2 hours to walk 6 miles but I am honored to dedicate those 2 hours in communication with my Creator.

You may be wondering what inspires me to keep going. Well, in addition to the visible signs of the weight loss, I also make a special effort to look good on my walk. I'm matched from head-to-toe. It really inspires me to keep going! People wave, at me, say, "Hi, you're doing it!" Sometimes, I get a few followers on the campus trail, just when I'm feeling the breath of life in my lungs.

You might be interested to know how to get started. Well, my schedule looks like this:

- My walk begins between 6:30 and 6:45 a.m.
- Before beginning the walk, stretch muscles.
- I take 20 deep breaths.

Why is stretching important?

There are several stretches and techniques that will improve the benefits of exercise walking, as well as helping to prevent injury.

Stretching before Walking

You should do **gentle stretching** to prepare the joints and muscles for the increased range of motion needed. It is important to take an easy five minute walk to warm up the muscles before stretching so they're not completely cold when stretching.

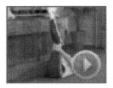

Hamstring Stretch Video

Discuss with a healthcare practitioner the best way to do stretches, and be sure to include the neck, arms, hips, upper and lower leg muscles (including the hamstring muscles in the back of the thigh), and Ankles.

- Start slowly. Map out a reasonable plan that you can commit to. Remember, consistency is the key to your success.
- Be sure to hydrate yourself.
- You're on your way. Be excited about the small bits of success you see. I guarantee those little glimpses will be just the motivation you need to catapult yourself to greatness.

As I also try to do some form of exercises at night, below are some suggestions for you:

- Floor exercises like leg raises and sit-ups. Feel free to implement your own personal choices.
- You may be wondering, what is a recumbent bicycle? A recumbent bicycle is a bicycle that places the rider in a laid-back reclining position. Because the position of the recumbent bicycle is more comfortable and supported, it offers a way for the de-conditioned individual to build up leg muscle strength. Many people, particularly the elderly and the obese, find upright cycle seats uncomfortable. Most recumbent bicycles feature a backrest

that can be helpful for riders who have spine injuries or who suffer from back pain. The handlebar is positioned at shoulder height, reducing pressure on shoulder joints and wrists.

http://healthyliving.azcentral.com

- An elliptical trainer or cross-trainer (also called an X-trainer) is a stationary exercise machine used to stimulate stair climbing, walking, or running without causing excessive pressure to the joints; hence, decreasing the risk of impact injuries. For this reason, people with some injuries can use an elliptical to stay fit, as the low impact affects them little.

http://en.wikipedia.org

To protect my replacement joints, my doctor advised me not to walk on a treadmill or to run, as it may damage my replaced joints. If you're concerned about whether or not to walk on a treadmill or to run, please consult your personal physician.

Step 4:
Revolutionize Your
Life by Walking

The American Heart Association says:

- Walking can lower risk of high blood pressure, high cholesterol and diabetes.
- The more people walked or ran each week, the more their heart benefits increased.

  http://newsroom.heart.org

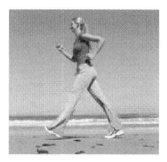

Regular exercise is good for us. Exercise keeps us healthy, helps us lose weight, and live longer. Of all forms of exercises, none are more popular than walking. And with good reason. Stride for stride, fitness experts agree that walking provides the most health and longevity benefits in the exercise arena. There are many reasons for this.

- Walking is low-impact. If we walk with proper form, we can eventually walk for long periods, which is even better for our metabolism and our cardiovascular system.

- "Chi walking is a technique that blends the health benefits of walking with core principles of T'ai Chi to deliver maximum physical, mental, and spiritual fitness. It involves a 5-step process to help you to learn to walk with excellent form?

- Walking can be done anywhere, even in a shopping mall or airport.

- Walking can be a great social activity where friends get fit together.

- Walking is cost-effective. You don't need a gym membership or fancy equipment, just a good pair of walking shoes.

- Nearly 80 million Americans consider themselves walkers, and this number is growing each year.

Despite this explosion, there is very little instruction available on how to walk properly. We all think we know how to walk in excellent form, but somehow we lose proper form, and our bodies become misaligned and imbalanced. From that, our joints become stiff. What must we do about that:

Get Aligned

- It promises to get you physically fit.
- Your form is totally dependent upon your posture.
- The efficiency of your walking form is in direct proportion to the quality of your posture.

- When your body weight is supported by your bones, ligaments, tendons ankles, hips, and shoulders, they are all connected in a straight line.
- When those dots are out of alignment even slightly, your muscles need to do the work of holding you upright.

One important principle that comes from T'ai Chi practice is called "needle and cotton." The needle represents the thin straight line of strength running vertically up through the body along the spine. It pulls energy into your center while letting go of tension in your extremities--your arms and legs so they can be soft and fluid, like cotton. You can then initiate all movement from that center line of strength.

- Begin by aligning your posture.
- Make sure your spine is long, tall and straight.
- If you maintain good posture in all your activities, not just walking, it will give your muscles a break and your brain a breath of fresh air.

Engage your Core

- The strongest part of your body is the one most involved in walking. Core strengthening is a very big topic in fitness circles. Your core muscles are the ones that are responsible for stabilizing your pelvic area in any activity, including sitting down. They hold your spine erect and help move your legs.
- To engage your core from a standing position, first set your feet hip-width apart and parallel.
- Relax your feet and soften your knees.

- Make your spine as long as you can by simply elongating your spine as though a string were attached to the crown of your head and was being pulled gently up to the sky.

- To engage your core, level your pelvis, place a hand on your belly, with your thumb at your naval and your fingers just above your pubic bone. Gently activate the pelvic muscles under your fingers so that it tilts.

- Imagine that your pelvis is a bowl of water; lift enough to keep the water from spilling from front or the back. If you are not sure which muscles to use, you'll find them easily if you laugh or cough.

Create Balance

Physical balance is essential for developing healthy, efficient walking form, and finding balance in our lives is an important aspect of healthy living. When you are physically balanced, it takes less work to support your body weight as well as create movement.

- When you are out of balance, your muscles have to do more work to compensate in walking, and you become tired more quickly.

- In ChiWalking, your body weight is always centered over your leading foot. That movement initiates from your center, and the bulk of the work is done by the core muscles, rather than your feet and legs having to reach out and pull you along.

- When you are physically balanced, you are not only more efficient in your walking; you are safer too, with much less potential for falling down or getting injured.

Make a Choice

Life is full of choices. We make thousands of them every day: what to wear, what to eat, which tasks to tackle first at work, and how we will respond to co-workers, kids or spouse.

Little choices can make a big difference because of their cumulative nature.

Take food for example-How we look or whether we carry extra pounds is not determined by one thing we eat, but rather by the accumulation of the dozens of food choices we make each day. This is compounded by days and weeks and years of our choices.

This step comes after we have gotten aligned, engaged our core, and created balance for a good reason. Many of the choices we make each day are so quick and often done unconsciously that if we are not in an aligned, balanced state, we can end up choosing poorly.

In ChiWalking, we choose to move forward in a different way than before, and that means to lead with our upper bodies, in balance over our stepping foot, rather than leading with our legs.

We choose which direction we are going before we start, so that all parts are moving in the same direction.

Move Forward

Now that you are aligned, centered in your engaged core, balanced over your feet, and have your destination in mind, you are ready to move forward. This is where the shoe leather meets the road, where you make that commitment to take a walk today and to lay out a plan for a weekly walking program toward good health and fitness.

- Keep moving forward, keep your posture straight, your core engaged, your upper body balanced over your lower body and your destination in mind. Moving forward sounds simple—because it is.

- Pay attention while completing the first four steps so that your forward movement has balance, purpose and direction.

  www.active.com/walking

  www.chiwalking.com

Step 5:
Good Walking Techniques are Key

Good Walking Techniques...

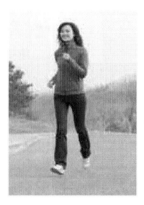

...make the difference between a good and a poor walking result. Good walking techniques keep you coming back because you feel great when you walk

The four elements of good walking technique include:

1. **Proper Posture**

    How you hold your body directly affects how comfortably and easily you walk. You breathe easier and avoid back pain.

    - Stand up straight.
    - Think and be tall. Don't arch your back.
    - Leaning forward or back puts extra strain on your

back muscles, and is counterproductive.

- Look straight ahead. Pick a spot to look at about 20 feet or more in front of you.
- Keep your chin parallel to the ground to reduce strain on your neck and back.
- Shrug once. Then let your shoulders fall slightly to the back and relax.
- Suck in your stomach. More!
- Tuck in your butt and rotate your hips forward slightly. This keeps you from arching your back.

2. Arm Motion

This motion lends power to your walking, helps balance your leg motion and results in 5-10% more calories burned while you're walking.

- Bend your elbows 90 degrees.
- Keep your hands loose and your fingers naturally curled and relaxed. Don't clench your fists. Clenching raises your blood pressure.
- Swing your arms fairly straight to the front and back as you walk. Don't let your hands cross the center point of your body
- Keep your elbows close to your body - don't go 'chicken wing'.
- On the forward motion, keep your hands lower than your breastbone. High arm motions don't help propel you.
- If the arm motion tires you at first, just do it for 5-10 minutes at a time then let your arms rest. Work up to a good, brisk arm movement for your entire walk.

3. Taking A Step

We believe you should know how to take a step but just to be sure...

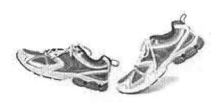

- Strike the ground first with your heel.
- Roll through the step from heel to toe.
- Push off with your toes.
- Bring back foot forward, strike ground with heel and repeat.

Shoe sole flexibility is important for comfortable walking. If your feet are slapping down rather than rolling through the step, your shoe soles are too stiff.

4. Walking Stride

- Take frequent, smaller steps. Your stride should be longer behind than out in front of your body.
- Don't extend your stride to increase speed (over-striding). This is inefficient and potentially harmful.
- Your back leg 'push' drives you forward. You get that power from your back leg as you push off the toe. This is the key to powerful and efficient walking. Your forward leg has no pushing power.
- Fast walkers train themselves to increase the number of steps per minute they take and make full use of the back stride.

www.50plus-fitness-walking-techniques.html

Step 6:
Defying the Odds

Well, I've shared my journey and quest to become organically healthy by instituting a program of walking which is sensible and yet provides the benefits you need to feel your best. Since instituting this walking program, I feel so much better about myself. My self-esteem has risen exponentially.

You see, I believe that age is just a number. I choose not to buy into the fact that I am a 67 year-old baby boomer. I want to continue to challenge myself to go to new heights of achievement. If I remain healthy, which I plan to do, I can only be hindered by myself and not by the voice of the naysayers and doubters, who I choose not to do.

My main intent and purpose for writing this book is to tell you that I'm really no different than you. What I've done to enhance my life is no different than what you're capable of doing to enhance your life. What separates the successful from those who don't even try is taking that first step. It's as simple as that!

Start slow and build is my suggestion for you. With each plateau of success you will be your own motivation for going to the next level. Others will compliment you, and you'll be gracious in accepting the accolades, but you will know that what you're doing is because of you and for you – no one else because you are the important one on your journey towards "60+ and Going Strong: Walking to a Healthier You."

I've made a genuine effort to make this book both useful and easily understood. Now, it's up to you to go and apply its illustrations and principles. You know what to do – just do it! Need serious motivation and guidance getting started, contact: www.rypenfitness.com

I salute you – you are all winners!

Step 7:
One Courageous Moment

Have you ever heard or perhaps used the phrase, "Money can buy many things but your health is not one of them?"

Unfortunately, once you're on a downward health spiral, it is sometimes difficult to stop it. It's like a train barreling down the tracks heading in the wrong direction and the conductor seems powerless to do anything about it. He knows the potential danger that looms, but when we're on that downward health spiral, we can also feel helpless. Being proactive about our health is always better than reacting to a devastating health crisis. There are some things we can do to help stave off the onset of serious diseases—yes, heart disease, cancer, diabetes, and high blood pressure can cause a lot of other diseases, such as kidney disease. Not to consider these health possibilities can cost you something you might not have thought of before.

We must dig deep and come up with the good stuff inside. Focus, persevere, and use the will to succeed. The worse thing we can do is to get stuck in that uncomfortable place and resign ourselves to defeat. The best thing we can do is to become our own cheerleader and do something for ourselves that brings good health.

Set goals, and then determine to meet those goals.

My double knee surgeries became my gift that kept on giving. I marveled at the plateaus I reached. I was so tired of taking pain medication and just knew there must be a better way – an organic way to better health. With my daily 6-mile, pain-free walking routine, I felt like the sky was the limit, and still do. I am now excited about exploring more opportunities for myself, which before were only thoughts. A whole new world has opened up for me. The great thing about my challenge is that it's not just for me; it's for anyone brave enough to get the diagnosis, then follow the proven method I've laid out, and watch with amazement the results!

As you reach a different plateau, thrive in that place, not just survive. Keep at it until you feel extraordinarily well. Now be well, act well, and encourage others to be well. When others see your new and sustained lifestyle, they will want, desire, and even strive to do the same, or emulate your efforts to some degree.

No one knows what lurks around life's corners but one thing is certain, if we treat our bodies well, then we can expect good, organic health to return to us.

Mine has been a fierce journey of patience, obedience to my inner self, and many tiny and major steps that brought me to the 6 mile-a-day that I now walk routinely.

It is with bubbling joy untold that brings me to this place of sharing my pain and triumph with you. It is not to boast of how great I am, but that YOU TOO can follow all 7 steps of power, and determination to bring you joy and organic health through perseverance to be bold and consistent with walking your way to health.

Your friend in organic health,

Janice M. Lauderdale

For more information

http://indiebestwriters.com

www.facebook.com/janicelauderdale

janmarielauderdale@gmail.com

www.wordpress.com/stats/jmlauderdale

BIOGRAPHY
Janice M. Lauderdale

Janice M. Lauderdale is wife to her husband Dennis for 40 years and has two grown successful children. After living through her own family's tragedy of elderly abuse, Ms. Lauderdale has written *"Wealth of the Wicked: an American Tragedy of Elderly Abuse,"* and, *"Baby Boomers and Seniors Free Yourself from Harm and Danger"* and has become an advocate for that segment of our society.

Lauderdale is also the author of *"60+ and Going Strong: Walking to a Healthier You"* which chronicles her triumphant journey through all the sadness she encountered while advocating on behalf of her 87-year old aunt who became the victim of elderly abuse at the hands of her nephew who took her to the bank, emptied out her safe deposit box of its contents, and under menace and duress had her sign a bogus living trust naming him as the sole beneficiary of her paid-for home.

Lauderdale's amazing journey to a balanced life centers around her focused efforts to get healthy after double knee replacement surgeries. This is a story that should interest all boomers and seniors and actually anyone else who has been dealt life's blows and made it back from the brink of disaster.

Her story serves as an inspiration and motivation to anyone contemplating joint replacement surgery and wondering what life will be like post-surgery. She is a real life example of what perseverance can do for those who believe and are willing to put in the hard work.

Six months after her bilateral knee surgeries, she embarked on a walking program which would lead her to finding balance in her life, and ultimately she saw great improvement in her health. She became her own motivation and believes anyone can do it.

Lauderdale has proved to the world that whatever you put your mind to, you can do. All it takes is making that first step!

Throw fear and all of its properties to the wind and declare that you will do whatever it takes to get to a better place – a balanced place with your health! You deserve to be free to live your life and to enjoy its beauty!

Regards,

Janice M. Lauderdale, author, motivational speaker, entrepreneur

http://Indiebestwriters.com

janmarielauderdale@gmail.com

www.twitter.com/janicemlauderda

www.facebook.com/janicemlauderdale

www.wordpress.com/stats/jmlauderdale

8370255R20023

Printed in Germany
by Amazon Distribution
GmbH, Leipzig